7

BASIC STEPS

TO

Successful
Fasting
& Prayer

Bill Bright

W9-BSB-556

NewLife
PUBLICATIONS
A MINISTRY OF CAMPUS CRUSADE FOR CHRIST

**Seven Basic Steps to
Successful Fasting and Prayer**

Published by
New*Life* Publications
A ministry of Campus Crusade for Christ
100 Sunport Lane
Orlando, FL 32809

Design and typesetting by Genesis Publications.

Printed in the United States of America.

ISBN 1-56399-073-3

Adapted from *The Coming Revival: America's Call to Fast, Pray, and "Seek God's Face,"* © 1995, Bill Bright. Published by New*Life* Publications.

As a personal policy, Bill Bright has never accepted honorariums or royalties for his personal use. Any royalties from his more than fifty books and thousands of articles are dedicated to helping fulfill the Great Commission, which has been his special burden for all of his Christian life.

CONTENTS

I believe the power of fasting as it relates to prayer is the spiritual atomic bomb that our Lord has given us to destroy the strongholds of evil and usher in a great revival and spiritual harvest around the world.

Increasingly I have been gripped with a growing sense of urgency to call upon God to send revival to our beloved country. In the spring and summer of 1994, I had a growing conviction that God wanted me to fast and pray for forty days for revival in America and for the fulfillment of the Great Commission in obedience to our Lord's command.

At first I questioned, "Is this truly God's call for me?" Forty days was a long time to go without solid food. But with each passing day, His call grew stronger and more clear. Finally, I was convinced. God was calling me to fast, and He would not make such a call without a specific reason or purpose. With this conviction, I entered my fast with excitement and expectancy mounting in my heart, praying, "Lord, what do You want me to do?"

I believe such a long fast was a sovereign call of God because of the magnitude of the sins of America and of the Church. The Lord impressed that upon my heart, as well as the urgent need to help accelerate the fulfillment of the Great Commission in this generation.

As I began my fast, I was not sure I could continue for forty days. But my confidence was in the Lord to help me. Each day His presence encouraged me to continue. The longer I fasted, the more I sensed the presence of the Lord. The Holy Spirit refreshed my soul and spirit, and I experienced the joy of the Lord as seldom before. Biblical truths leaped at me from the pages of God's Word. My faith soared as I humbled myself and cried out to God and rejoiced in His presence.

This proved to be the most important forty days of my life. As I waited upon the Lord, the Holy Spirit gave me the assurance that America and much of the world will, before the end of the year 2000, experience a great spiritual awakening. This divine visit from heaven will kindle the greatest spiritual harvest in the history of the Church. But before God comes in revival power, the Holy Spirit will call millions of God's people to repent, fast, and pray in the spirit of 2 Chronicles 7:14:

> *If my people, who are called by my name, will humble themselves and pray and seek my face and turn from their wicked ways, then will I hear from heaven and will forgive their sin and will heal their land.*

The scope of this revival depends on how believers in America and the rest of the world respond to this call. I have spent fifty years studying God's Word and listening to His voice, and His message could not have been more clear.

This handy reference guide, *Seven Basic Steps to Successful Fasting and Prayer*, will help make your time with the Lord more spiritually rewarding. I encourage you to keep it with you during your fast and refer to it often because it gives easy-to-follow suggestions on how to begin your fast, what to do while you fast, and how to end your fast properly.

During my forty-day fast, God impressed me to pray that two million Christians in North America will fast for forty days by the end of the year 2000, and pray for national and worldwide revival and for the fulfillment of the Great Commission. I urge you to prayerfully consider this challenge.

Before you fast, I encourage you to read my book, *The Coming Revival: America's Call to Fast, Pray, and "Seek God's Face."* It will help equip you for the coming spiritual awakening.

Bill Bright

HOW TO BEGIN YOUR FAST

How you begin and conduct your fast will largely determine your success. By following these seven basic steps to fasting, you will make your time with the Lord more meaningful and spiritually rewarding.

STEP 1 **Set Your Objective**

Why are you fasting? Is it for spiritual renewal, for guidance, for healing, for the resolution of problems, for special grace to handle a difficult situation? Ask the Holy Spirit to clarify His leading and objectives for your prayer fast. This will enable you to pray more specifically and strategically.

Through fasting and prayer we humble ourselves before God so the Holy Spirit will stir our souls, awaken our churches, and heal our land according to 2 Chronicles 7:14. Make this a priority in your fasting.

STEP 2 **Make Your Commitment**

Pray about the kind of fast you should undertake. Jesus implied that all of His followers should fast (Matthew 6:16–18; 9:14,15). For Him it was a matter of *when* believers would fast, not *if* they would do it. Before you fast, decide the following up front:

- How long you will fast—one meal, one day, a week, several weeks, forty days (Beginners should start slowly, building up to longer fasts.)

- The type of fast God wants you to undertake (such as water only, or water and juices; what kinds of juices you will drink and how often)

- What physical or social activities you will restrict

- How much time each day you will devote to prayer and God's Word

Making these commitments ahead of time will help you sustain your fast when physical temptations and life's pressures tempt you to abandon it.

STEP 3 Prepare Yourself Spiritually

The very foundation of fasting and prayer is repentance. Unconfessed sin will hinder your prayers. Here are several things you can do to prepare your heart:

- Ask God to help you make a comprehensive list of your sins.

- Confess every sin that the Holy Spirit calls to your remembrance and accept God's forgiveness (1 John 1:9).

- Seek forgiveness from all whom you have offended, and forgive all who have hurt you (Mark 11:25; Luke 11:4; 17:3,4).
- Make restitution as the Holy Spirit leads you.
- Ask God to fill you with His Holy Spirit according to His *command* in Ephesians 5:18 and His *promise* in 1 John 5:14,15.
- Surrender your life fully to Jesus Christ as your Lord and Master; refuse to obey your worldly nature (Romans 12:1,2).
- Meditate on the attributes of God, His love, sovereignty, power, wisdom, faithfulness, grace, compassion, and others (Psalm 48:9,10; 103:1–8,11–13).
- Begin your time of fasting and prayer with an expectant heart (Hebrews 11:6).
- Do not underestimate spiritual opposition. Satan sometimes intensifies the natural battle between body and spirit (Galatians 5:16,17).

STEP 4 · Prepare Yourself Physically

Fasting requires reasonable precautions. Consult your physician first, especially if you take prescription medication or have a chronic ailment. Some persons should never fast without professional supervision.

Physical preparation makes the drastic change in your eating routine a little easier so that you can turn your full attention to the Lord in prayer.

- Do not rush into your fast.
- Prepare your body. Eat smaller meals before starting a fast. Avoid high-fat and sugary foods.
- Eat raw fruit and vegetables for two days before starting a fast.

WHILE YOU FAST

Your time of fasting and prayer has come. You are abstaining from all solid foods and have begun to seek the Lord. Here are some helpful suggestions to consider:

- Avoid drugs, even natural herbal drugs and homeopathic remedies. Medication should be withdrawn only with your physician's supervision.
- Limit your activity.
- Exercise only moderately. Walk one to three miles each day if convenient and comfortable.
- Rest as much as your schedule will permit.

- Prepare yourself for temporary mental discomforts, such as impatience, crankiness, and anxiety.

- Expect some physical discomforts, especially on the second day. You may have fleeting hunger pains, dizziness, or the "blahs." Withdrawal from caffeine and sugar may cause headaches. Physical annoyances may also include weakness, tiredness, or sleeplessness.

The first two or three days are usually the hardest. As you continue to fast, you will likely experience a sense of well-being both physically and spiritually. However, should you feel hunger pains, increase your liquid intake.

STEP 5 Put Yourself on a Schedule

For maximum spiritual benefit, set aside ample time to be alone with the Lord. Listen for His leading. The more time you spend with Him, the more meaningful your fast will be.

Morning

- Begin your day in praise and worship.
- Read and meditate on God's Word, preferably on your knees.

- Invite the Holy Spirit to work in you to will and to do His good pleasure according to Philippians 2:13.
- Invite God to use you. Ask Him to show you how to influence your world, your family, your church, your community, your country, and beyond.
- Pray for His vision for your life and empowerment to do His will.

Noon
- Return to prayer and God's Word.
- Take a short prayer walk.
- Spend time in intercessory prayer for your community's and nation's leaders, for the world's unreached millions, for your family or special needs.

Evening
- Get alone for an unhurried time of "seeking His face."
- If others are fasting with you, meet together for prayer.
- Avoid television or any other distraction that may dampen your spiritual focus.

When possible, begin and end each day on your knees with your spouse for a brief time of praise and thanksgiving to God. Longer periods of time with our Lord in prayer and study of His Word are often better spent alone.

A dietary routine is vital as well. Dr. Julio C. Ruibal—nutritionist, pastor, and specialist in fasting and prayer—suggests a daily schedule and list of juices you may find useful and satisfying. Modify this schedule and the drinks you take to suit your circumstances and tastes.

5 a.m. – 8 a.m.

Fruit juices, preferably freshly squeezed or blended and diluted in 50 percent distilled water if the fruit is acid. Apple, pear, grapefruit, papaya, watermelon, or other fruit juices are generally preferred. If you cannot do your own juicing, buy juices without sugar or additives.

10:30 a.m. – noon

Fresh vegetable juice made from lettuce, celery, and carrots in three equal parts.

2:30 p.m. – 4 p.m.

Herb tea with a drop of honey. Avoid black tea or any tea with caffeine.

6 p.m. – 8:30 p.m.

Broth made from boiling potatoes, celery, and carrots with no salt. After boiling about half an hour, pour the water into a container and drink it.

Tips on Juice Fasting

- Drinking fruit juice will decrease your hunger pains and give you some natural sugar energy. The taste and lift will motivate and strengthen you to continue.

- The best juices are made from fresh watermelon, lemons, grapes, apples, cabbage, beets, carrots, celery, or leafy green vegetables. In cold weather, you may enjoy warm vegetable broth.

- Mix acidic juices (orange, tomato) with water for your stomach's sake.

- Avoid caffeinated drinks. And avoid chewing gum or mints, even if your breath is bad. They stimulate digestive action in your stomach.

BREAKING YOUR FAST

When your designated time for fasting is finished, you will begin to eat again. But how you break your fast is extremely important for your physical and spiritual well-being.

STEP 6 **End Your Fast Gradually**
Begin eating gradually. Do not eat solid foods immediately after your fast. Suddenly reintroducing solid food to your stomach and digestive tract will likely have

negative, even dangerous, consequences. Try several smaller meals or snacks each day. If you end your fast gradually, the beneficial physical and spiritual effects will result in continued good health.

Here are some suggestions to help you end your fast properly:

- Break an extended water fast with fruit such as watermelon.
- While continuing to drink fruit or vegetable juices, add the following:

First day: Add a raw salad.

Second day: Add baked or boiled potato, no butter or seasoning.

Third day: Add a steamed vegetable.

Thereafter: Begin to reintroduce your normal diet.

- Gradually return to regular eating with several small snacks during the first few days. Start with a little soup and fresh fruits such as watermelon and cantaloupe. Advance to a few tablespoons of solid foods such as raw fruits and vegetables or a raw salad and baked potato.

STEP 7 — Expect Results

If you sincerely humble yourself before the Lord, repent, pray, and seek God's face; if you consistently meditate on His Word, you will experience a heightened awareness of His presence (John 14:21). The Lord will give you fresh, new spiritual insights. Your confidence and faith in God will be strengthened. You will feel mentally, spiritually, and physically refreshed. You will see answers to your prayers.

A single fast, however, is not a spiritual cure-all. Just as we need fresh infillings of the Holy Spirit daily, we also need new times of fasting before God. A 24-hour fast each week has been greatly rewarding to many Christians.

It takes time to build your spiritual fasting muscles. If you fail to make it through your first fast, do not be discouraged. You may have tried to fast too long the first time out, or you may need to strengthen your understanding and resolve. As soon as possible, undertake another fast until you do succeed. God will honor you for your faithfulness.

I encourage you to join me in fasting and prayer again and again until we truly experience revival in our homes, our churches, our beloved nation, and throughout the world.

How to Experience and Maintain Personal Revival

1. Ask the Holy Spirit to reveal any unconfessed sin in your life.

2. Seek forgiveness from all whom you have offended, and forgive all who have hurt you. Make restitution where God leads.

3. Examine your motives in every word and deed. Ask the Lord to search and cleanse your heart daily.

4. Ask the Holy Spirit to guard your walk against complacency and mediocrity.

5. Praise and give thanks to God continually in all ways on all days, regardless of your circumstances.

6. Refuse to obey your carnal (worldly) nature (Galatians 5:16,17).

7. Surrender your life to Jesus Christ as your Savior and Lord. Develop utter dependence on Him with total submission and humility.

8. Study the attributes of God.

9. Hunger and thirst after righteousness (Matthew 5:6).

10. Love God with all of your heart, soul, and mind (Matthew 22:37).

11. Appropriate the continual fullness and control of the Holy Spirit by faith on the basis of God's *command* (Ephesians 5:18) and *promise* (1 John 5:14,15).

12. Read, study, meditate on, and memorize God's holy, inspired, inerrant Word daily (Colossians 3:16).

13. Pray without ceasing (1 Thessalonians 5:17).

14. Fast and pray one 24-hour period each week. Prayerfully consider becoming one of the two million Christians who will fast for forty days before the end of the year 2000.

15. Seek to share Christ daily as a way of life.

16. Determine to live a holy, godly life of obedience and faith.

17. Start or join a home or church Bible study group that emphasizes revival and a holy life.

Six Vital Questions About Prayer

Q What Is Prayer?

Simply put, prayer is communicating with God. Real prayer is expressing our devotion to our heavenly Father, inviting Him to talk to us as we talk to Him.

Q Who Can Pray?

Anyone can pray, but only those who walk in faith and obedience to Christ can expect to receive answers to their prayers.

Contact with God begins when we receive Jesus into our lives as Savior and Lord (John 14:6). Praying with a clean heart is also vital to successful prayer. We cannot expect God to answer our prayers if there is any unconfessed sin in our life or if we are harboring an unforgiving spirit (Psalm 66:18; Mark 11:25). For God to answer our prayers, we must have a believing heart and ask according to His will (Matthew 9:29; 21:22; 1 John 5:14,15).

Q Why Are We to Pray?

God's Word commands us to pray (Luke 18:1; Acts 6:4; Mark 14:38; Philippians 4:6; Colossians 4:2; 1 Timothy 2:1,2).

We pray to have fellowship with God, receive spiritual nurture and strength to live a victorious life, and maintain boldness for a vital witness for Christ.

Prayer releases God's great power to change the course of nature, people, and nations.

Q To Whom Do We Pray?

We pray to the Father in the name of the Lord Jesus Christ through the ministry of the Holy Spirit. When we pray to the Father, our prayers are accepted by Jesus Christ and interpreted to God the Father by the Holy Spirit (Romans 8:26,27,34).

Q When Should We Pray?

God's Word commands us to "Pray continually" (1 Thessalonians 5:17). We can be in prayer throughout the day, expressing and demonstrating our devotion to God as we go about our daily tasks.

It is not always necessary to be on our knees, or even in a quiet room to pray. God want us to be in touch with Him constantly wherever we are. We can pray in the car, while washing the dishes, or while walking down the street.

Q What Should We Include in Our Prayers?

Although prayer cannot be reduced to a formula, certain basic elements should be included in our communication with God: *Adoration, Confession, Thanksgiving, Supplication* (ACTS).

A—*Adoration*

To adore God is to worship and praise Him, to honor and exalt Him in our heart and mind and with our lips.

C—*Confession*

When our discipline of prayer begins with adoration, the Holy Spirit has opportunity to reveal any sin in our life that needs to be confessed.

T—*Thanksgiving*

An attitude of thanksgiving to God, for who He is and for the benefits we enjoy because we belong to Him, enables us to recognize that He controls all things—not just the blessings, but the problems and adversities as well. As we approach God with a thankful heart, He becomes strong on our behalf.

S—*Supplication*

Supplication includes petition for our own needs and intercession for others. Pray that your inner person may be renewed, always sensitive to and empowered by the Holy Spirit. Pray for others—your spouse, your children, your parents, neighbors, and friends; our nation and those in authority over us. Pray for the salvation of souls, for a daily opportunity to introduce others to Christ and to the ministry of the Holy Spirit, and for the fulfillment of the Great Commission.

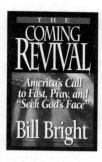

Our nation is in a moral free-fall and the Church for the most part is spiritually impotent. What can we do to stop the tragic decline? This book gives the startling answer!

Easy-to-read. The thoughts are fresh. The challenge is compelling. (224 pp., $9.99)

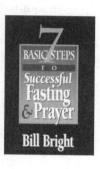

This handy reference guide to fasting and prayer is available alone or as a companion to *The Coming Revival*. (24 pp., $4.95 pkg. 5)

RESPONSE FORM

☐ Dr. Bright, I want to be one of the two million people who will join you in forty days of fasting and prayer for revival.

☐ Please send me information on quantity discounts for *The Coming Revival* and *Seven Basic Steps to Successful Fasting and Prayer* to give to my pastor, church, loved ones, and friends.

☐ Please inform me of other materials on how I can be filled with the Holy Spirit and be more effective in my prayer and Christian witness.

NAME

ADDRESS

CITY

STATE   ZIP

(   )

PHONE

Please check the appropriate box(es) and mail this form in an envelope to:

> Bill Bright
> Campus Crusade for Christ
> P.O. Box 593684
> Orlando, FL 32859